The Power of Japanese Red Reishi:
The Real Magic Mushroom™

Reverse biological aging and enhance immunity
with the help of one of nature's most powerful
medicinal mushrooms.

Brad J. King and Dr. Meg Jordan

Published in Canada by
World Health Publishing Inc.

Cover, Text design and typesetting by Kato Design Ltd
Illustrations by Robert Browne and Florence Ng

Printed in China by Leanne Publishing Inc.

*Permission to use the phrase, "real magic mushroom",
have been authorized by Nikkei (Canada) Marketing Ltd, Canada."*

TABLE OF CONTENTS

INTRODUCTION.. 3
    Medicinal Mushrooms 10
    A Short History of Reishi 15

CHAPTER ONE
    The Secret to Aging Well 19
    Our Ever Changing Body 21
    The Metabolic States 22
    Red Reishi – Its Role as an Adaptogen 26
    A Healthy Liver = A Healthier Body 29
    Your Liver and Weight Control 31

CHAPTER TWO
    Battle Stress 35
    The Quest for Energy 43

CHAPTER THREE
    Maintaining Immunity as we Age............................. 47
    Enhancing Immunity – A Key to Successful Aging....... 54
    The Secret Weapon – Japanese Red Reishi................. 57
    Monitoring and Repairing the Immune System 62
    Diabetes – the Obesity Connection 65
    Anti-inflammatory Effects 68
    Cardiovascular Benefits 69
    Cancer Support 73
    Frequently Asked Questions 76
    Quality Matters – Choosing the Right Red Reishi 77
    Common Growing Techniques 80
    Conclusion 91

INTRODUCTION

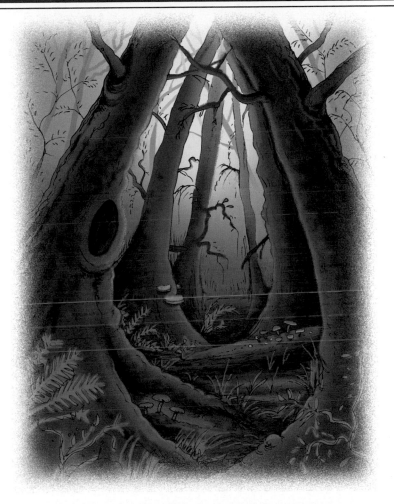

A mystery that dwells deep in the forest offers a potential healing balm for many of today's most devastating diseases, especially cancer, which has recently inched past heart disease as the chief killer of our time.

When you hike on trails shaded by towering trees, the soil moist and soft underfoot, you can spot large fan-shaped mushrooms attached to felled logs. Here in this quiet kingdom the seamless cycle of life is abundantly clear. Persistent and tenacious, these fungi factories slowly digest decaying matter, making way for new life.

It is phenomenal to think that nothing in nature is wasted, and life is continually recycled. The ability of certain mushrooms to transform dead cells into life-enhancing compounds is a miraculous event, and may provide a clue about their immune enhancing and anti-cancer properties.

In a laboratory experiment, a stubborn tumor suddenly shrinks as a once dormant immune system suddenly springs into action, coordinating a series of events which culminate in what many today would deem "a miracle". Yet the only so-called miracle happening here is the body's immune system being "activated" or "turned-on", to do a job it was always designed to do. The fact remains – especially as we get older – we can sometimes use a little push in the right direction. In this case, the push comes from a high proportion of specialized plant compounds found in a single mushroom extract.

Exciting scientific discoveries regarding medical mushrooms (Red Reishi, shiitake, cordyceps, maitake) over the past 30 years have been confirming what herbalists and traditional Chinese medicine doctors have purported for centuries. The ability of these medicinal mushrooms to transform dead matter into life-enhancing miracle compounds allows them to provide perhaps, the most potent immune-enhancing and anti-cancer properties known on earth.

As researchers, it is our job (and passion) to sift through the research and bring to light the most effective, safe and natural approaches to maintaining optimal health. Many of these approaches come from the plant kingdom (including almost 30 percent of prescription meds), in which literally thousands of health enhancing, side-effect free compounds have already been discovered. We can honestly say that out of hundreds of nutritional wonders we have looked at, written about and personally consumed over the years, only a handful stand out as true miracles of nature. The problem is that once these incredible health enhancing nutrients are brought to the public, too many times their healing properties are greatly reduced by ineffective or inconsistent cultivation, extraction and/or manufacturing practices.

Red Reishi (Ganoderma lucidum) stands out as the true monarch of the forest, long hailed for its medicinal qualities by physicians serving emperors and royal dynasties in Japan and China for thousands of years.

Red Reishi mushrooms are rare in the wild, and require the utmost care when being cultivated and having their medicinal properties extracted. The end result of extraction is Red Reishi essence in its most bio-available form, especially if it has been grown on aged logs and manufactured by the Japanese in a highly controlled environment (as you will learn later in this book).

As a potent immune modulator – a substance that supports optimal immune health – Red Reishi essence can be safely taken on a daily basis, is non-toxic, and improves overall health and longevity. It provides benefits for the immune system, cardiovascular system, liver protection, metabolism, blood sugar balance, and reduces the damaging effects of stress and chronic inflammation. Most people also report feeling more energetic, less stressed out and that they are able to concentrate better.

But it is the cancer-treating applications that have most of us curious. Integrative health experts predict that medicinal mushrooms will play an increasingly important role as a cancer-preventive, as anti-tumor agents, and as adjunctive support for those undergoing chemotherapy since medicinal mushrooms help reduce the toxic effects of conventional therapy.

We are excited by what we have uncovered regarding the amazing and numerous health benefits associated with Red Reishi. We also can't wait to share this health enhancing information with you. So what are you waiting for? Turn the page and let's get started…

COPING WITH OUR CRAZY WORLD
Life is making us old.

Work stress, family stress, stress from pollution, poor eating habits; these all take a toll on our bodies, wearing us down and causing us to age much more quickly than we should. In fact, according to Dr. Robert Sapolsky, Professor of Biological Sciences at Stanford University, "In many ways, aging can be defined as the progressive loss of the ability to deal with stress."

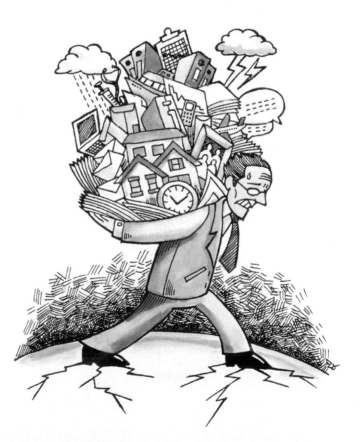

Stress is like an annoying little construction worker with a hammer, chipping away at our body's foundation. We are only as strong as our ability to maintain a healthy foundation, and once the foundation is weakened, we lose the ability to stay healthy. You know what this feels like: short bouts of colds, flu, aching joints, etc., followed by longer and longer ones. Soon, illness becomes the norm; we've begun to break down. And we begin to feel old - as this attack on our foundation continues - regardless of how many candles were actually on our last birthday cake.

The bottom line is that most of us just don't take care of ourselves. Oh sure, we have good intentions, but there never seems to be enough time – time to work out, time to rest, time to eat nutrient rich foods, time to do the things that boost our energy. But if right now, by picking up this book, you've decided to make a change, to feel better, to improve your overall well-being, then we invite you to take a moment to reflect on the wisdom of the past. To a time when there were no electronic gadgets, no traffic jams and no pollution. What if we told you that there was an ancient and powerful herb that could help you to cope with the stress (and distress) in your life, and it's something that has been used safely since ancient times? What if we told you that this very herb could help enhance your energy levels and take your health to the next level?

Help is on the Way...

It's called the Red Reishi mushroom. You probably haven't heard much about it, because for a long time it was very hard to find. In fact, for thousands of years, Red Reishi was found only in the high, remote mountains of China because of its very specific growing requirements of sunshine, temperature, and humidity. It was exceedingly rare. Known as the "King of Herbs", only the very rich and powerful could afford to send servants out to isolated and often treacherous locations to search for it.

Now, Red Reishi is finally available here in North America. Thanks to the years of dedicated study by many world-renowned researchers, we now understand how to nurture and grow this important herb, and how to concentrate all of its health-giving properties in essence form.

In this book, you'll see why health practitioners the world over are convinced that supplements derived from mushrooms, and Japanese Red Reishi in particular, can significantly improve your mind, body, and spirit as well as your overall well-being. You'll learn how Japanese Red Reishi is the best at enhancing your ability to deal with many of life's insults by boosting your immune system. We'll show you why ...read on!

MEDICINAL MUSHROOMS

Mushrooms have been respected for their healing properties for thousands of years. That's simply because they are very effective at treating some illnesses. Many herbs once ignored by Western medicine are now either accepted to be effective treatment, or have attracted enough interest to be under serious consideration in laboratories all over the world. As examples, these are some of the many plants with proven benefits; as you will see, Japanese Red Reishi is the leader of the pack.

Cordyceps

 Also called the "caterpillar fungus" for its primary host (it infects caterpillars and kills them), Cordyceps has a long history of use in Chinese medicine. Its traditional roles have been restorative, improving the quality of life, and increasing energy and longevity.

While most of the Cordyceps research has been conducted in China, published studies in Europe and elsewhere indicate that the fungus may have some potentially useful properties. A Korean study of a related species of Cordyceps shows that it has components that may inhibit coagulation (blood clot formation), making it potentially beneficial in stroke and heart attack prevention, very much like what daily Aspirin is recommended for, but without the gastrointestinal side effects. A hot water extract of the fungus appeared to stimulate the immune system. Other studies have reported that Cordyceps may be useful in treating Hepatitis B.

Researchers from Thailand reported that a variety of Cordyceps might have value in the treatment of malaria, while other researchers concluded that Cordyceps might be promising as a possible aid for fatigue, stress, heart health, lung function, and toxin exposure. One study looked at herbs used as performance enhancers (to improve exercise and athletic performance) and was unable to validate Cordyceps value for this purpose. While Cordyceps has many healing properties, Red Reishi, still has more.

Maitake

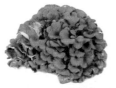

The name Maitake means "dancing mushroom". Also called "hen of the woods", and "sheep's head", Maitake is naturally found in the northeastern part of Japan and North America, and is prized in traditional Chinese and Japanese herbology as an adaptogen. It also contains Beta-glucans, which as you will learn are useful in enhancing the immune system. Maitake is rich in minerals (K, Ca, Mg), various vitamins (B2, D2, and Niacin), fibre, and amino acids. Most people find its taste appealing, but the mushroom has been known to cause allergic reactions in some people.

Shiitake

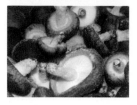

Shiitake mushrooms have been researched for their medicinal benefits, most notably their anti-tumor properties in laboratory mice. These studies have also identified the Polysaccharide lentinan, as the active compound responsible for its anti-tumor effects. Shiitake may activate specialized immune cells called macrophages, as well as increase other immune enhancers like Interleukin-1 production, proliferation of B lymphocytes and antibody production.

Extracts from shiitake mushrooms have also been researched for many other immunological benefits, ranging from anti-viral properties to possible treatments for allergies, as well as arthritis.

Lentionine, a key flavour compound of shiitake, also inhibits platelet aggregation, the process by which blood cells clump together, so it is a promising treatment for blood clots in veins and arteries (thrombosis), working as an agent to prevent cardiovascular events, as well as reducing the incidences of certain cancers.

Shiitake are also one of a few known natural sources of vegan and kosher vitamin D (vitamin D2).

Coriolus

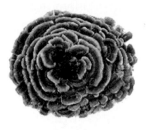

In China, Coriolus is known as "Yun zhi", or the "cloud mushroom". In Japan it is called "Kawaratake", or "mushroom by the river". In traditional herbalism, hot water extracts of Coriolus were used to dispel dampness, reduce phlegm, treat pulmonary infections, and to support liver health. The Ming dynasty edition of the Materia Media states, "The black and green Yun zhi are beneficial to one's spirit and vital energy, and strengthen one's tendon and bone. If Yun zhi is taken for a long time, it will make one vigorous and live long."

In Japan these mushrooms are also highly prized and sought after by people suffering from a variety of chronic conditions. In fact, it was a neighbor's success in using Coriolus for stomach cancer that first caught the attention of a scientist that worked for the Japanese company Kureha Chemicals, and subsequently launched the research and development of what came to be known as PSK. PSK (Polysaccharide Krestin) is an approved anti-cancer drug with 20 years of research in Japan.

Wood Ear

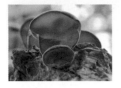

Widely respected in the Orient for its taste, the Wood Ear mushroom is also believed to have medicinal benefits. Thought by many to prevent heart disease and contain anticoagulant-type substances, acting like blood thinners that may prevent blood clots with an effect similar to that of aspirin.

Polyporus

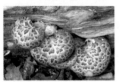

Polyporus mushrooms are used in cases of edema, cloudy urination, burning urination, vaginal discharge, diarrhea, and jaundice.

Mushrooms
research and time proven

As you are now aware, medicinal mushrooms—many of which have been used for centuries—are scientifically documented to help in the treatment of many disorders. While it is true that there are a number of mushroom products on the market, it has been known for thousands of years that **Red Reishi is the most effective**. Health-giving compounds are most highly concentrated in Red Reishi, with active ingredients for vitality, immune support, and as we will see, even cancer prevention and treatment.

A SHORT HISTORY OF REISHI

In ancient times, it was said that if you discovered Reishi growing in the forest, you must keep the secret even from your closest relative – it was that highly regarded.

Shennong was a brave man. He was Emperor of China four thousand years ago, and wrote his "Divine Farmers Herb Root Classic"– the very first Traditional Chinese Medicine pharmacopeia – 'way back around 2730BC. "Brave", because legend has it that he personally consumed 365 plants, and evaluated them for the range of illnesses they treated, how effective they were, and the number of side effects they had (i.e., were they poisonous!?). After he'd done all the tasting and testing - and recovered from the poisonous ones - he used what he'd learned to place them in one of three classes: "Fair", "Average", and "Superior". Red Reishi was the Big Winner! In fact, Shennong was so impressed with what he learned about Red Reishi, that he awarded it the honour of being the best of the "Superior" plants. He judged it to be even better than the fabled Ginseng root in effectiveness, range of illnesses that it combatted, and absence of side effects.

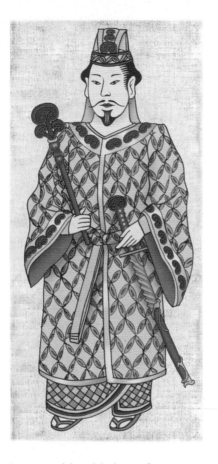

Reishi soon became the most sought after medicinal herb in Eastern medicine. Its level of importance in Chinese Medicine is expressed in the many ways it has been incorporated into Oriental art and culture. Reishi was depicted in paintings, embroideries, buildings, sculptures, and carvings of the gods and immortals, as a symbol of divinity and longevity. Reishi was a favorite ornamental design feature of the royalty and the wealthy, sometimes as much for good luck as for its actual health benefits. Pictures of Reishi can still be seen everywhere in the Forbidden City and the Summer Palace in Beijing, evidence of its high status in ancient Chinese society. Even the traditional scepter of the emperors of China was a stylized Reishi, called a Ru Yi. (the first scepter was more than likely a real Reishi!).

Traditionally in China, Reishi was considered to be among the most valuable possessions a new bride could bring into a marriage because of its many benefits.

There are many varieties of Reishi mushrooms found in

nature—over 2000 to be exact! Of all these varieties, a small number have been shown to have potent medicinal benefits. These medicinal mushrooms are further classified by their colour: Black, Blue, White, Yellow, Purple or Red. Of these varieties, **Red Reishi** is by far the most effective at improving the body's ability to cope with stress, disease, and immune system breakdown. This is because it has the highest concentration of powerful, plant-kingdom medicinal agents, called phytonutrients.

But not all Red Reishi products are created equal in quality and strength - not by a long shot. There are big differences in the way the mushrooms are grown and processed, and these differences can have a huge impact on the potency of the product that ends up on the store shelf. One of the major factors, for instance, is the quality of the Red Reishi strain that is used to begin the process. Low quality strains will have low concentrations of the active nutrients, and therefore be less effective. Another factor is the producers' willingness to wait until the mushroom is fully mature before harvesting it. Some harvest immature plants, which also have low concentrations of the active components, and are therefore much less potent.

For maximum benefits, and to ensure the highest quality Red Reishi, only Japanese variety Red Reishi should be purchased. This is due to the unsurpassed growing and extracting practices of Japanese Red Reishi. In fact, there is an actual Red Reishi policing organization called The Japan Reishi Association, that allows only those that adhere to the strictest of standards, to bare their association's hologram on finished products (more on this later).

RED REISHI...
What Can It Do For Me?

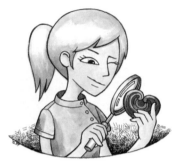

Red Reishi has been used with safety and great success for thousands of years, yet it has only been commercially cultivated for about 25 years. Has it been worth the wait? Absolutely!

Research indicates that Red Reishi can strengthen your body's response to disease-causing processes and bring your body's functions back to normal (rebuild and strengthen the foundation). We don't claim that Red Reishi cures all illnesses (or any for that matter), but research clearly indicates that taking it every day can play a big role in disease prevention by improving your overall ability to cope with life's stresses – mental, physical and environmental. We encourage you to make Red Reishi an important part of your health and wellness routine.

Before we explain how Red Reishi works, let's look at the way our body handles aging and stress. Some of what follows might be a little technical, but we think that you should be properly informed about anything that claims to be as important as Red Reishi, so please read on…you'll see why we're so excited about the many health benefits of this amazing plant.

CHAPTER ONE

THE SECRET TO AGING WELL

Remember When?

DO YOU REMEMBER HOW YOU FELT LIKE WHEN YOU were really young? If you're like most of us, you took your excess energy for granted. Looking, feeling and performing great were things that just happened – you 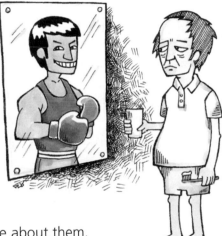 didn't have to think twice about them. Everything worked so well because your body invested a lot of time and energy on repairs. Cuts, scrapes, sunburn, infections all healed very quickly. It was as if you had a full-time mechanic on the premises.

If you take time to watch a child, you will soon understand the miracle of life – life in the truest sense of the word. Children live every moment to the fullest. They contain the essential mechanics of life. They are in a constant state of rebuilding and renewing their bodies as they are always in perfect balance with their internal systems. A child is the most incredible self-repairing organism of all.

Even as adults, our bodies are in a constant mode of regeneration, or at least they should be. The cells that comprise our organs, the bones that frame them, the muscles that hold up the frame, and the skin that covers the structures, are all being renewed at an astonishing rate when we are young and vital. When we're healthy, we can rebuild and replace our structures at the rate of almost 200 million cells a minute, which means nearly 300 billion, repaired, replaced and replenished cells per day. In a sense, we wake up as a different person each morning!

But our ability to rebuild our cells doesn't necessarily depend on how old we are in years - called our "chronological age", and yes, you can stop crying every time you see those birthday candles on your cake. What matters most is how our body— and the cells that comprise it—is aging, called our "biological age". If we take advantage of every opportunity to strengthen our bodies by eating well and taking the proper supplements, exercising, and getting enough sleep, then biological aging will happen as slowly as possible. This is also called "optimal aging" or "healthy longevity", as opposed to "premature aging" which is what happens when we don't take care of our bodies. You can have healthy longevity; it's all about maintaining balance within the body's internal systems.

OUR EVER CHANGING BODY

The Amazing Machine

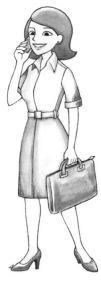

WE'VE ALL HEARD THE TERM "METABO-LISM". THAT JUST refers to the way our body constantly grows, repairs, reproduces cells, and reacts to the environment. Everything it does requires chemical reactions of one kind or another. For example, the food you eat must be broken down into individual or groups of components, also referred to as building blocks, before your body can use it, and these building blocks are used to create other compounds that your body needs. Our metabolism is the sum of all of the huge number of chemical reactions that take place, 24 hours a day, within your body (yes, even while you are fast asleep and dreaming). Depending on the circumstances, your metabolism shifts its focus from time to time to "concentrate" on specific parts of the metabolic process; specific groups of chemical reactions. We refer to these shifts as changes in "the metabolic state". The human body is constantly going through various metabolic states during the day and night. It's through these various states that biological aging makes its biggest impact.

THE METABOLIC STATES

The Anabolic State

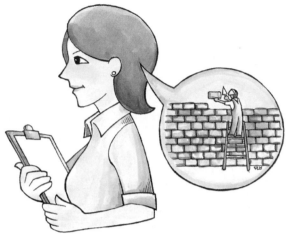

THE WORD "ANABOLIC" JUST MEANS, "TO BUILD UP". The anabolic state of health is where the cells of your body are constantly renewing and rebuilding themselves. In the anabolic state, all of your body's systems are in a constant mode of renewal and rebuilding.

This process of renewal is controlled by our anabolic metabolism, the system through which our 100 trillion cells rebuild, replenish and repair themselves. In a sense, anabolic metabolism is our repair budget. The bigger the budget, the more we can afford the repair bills. When we're young and healthy, our repair budget is extremely high. Our body regenerates its cells with incredible speed and efficiency. But as we get older and neglect to make the healthy choices our bodies need us to make – the budget gets smaller, the repair bills go unpaid, and we start to break down. Once this delicate balance is interrupted, we move into the catabolic state.

The Catabolic State

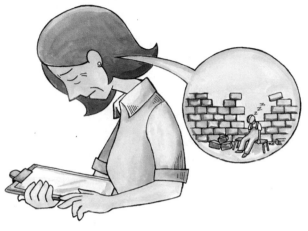

The word "catabolic" means to "break down". The catabolic state—in longevity research—is when your repair mechanisms start to slow down and become out of balance with the body's destructive mechanisms. This catabolic process depletes the body systems, especially the bones and muscles. Thus health and vitality begin to degenerate regardless of age. Many longevity researchers now believe that premature aging really begins the day your body breaks down faster than it can rebuild itself. This is when your foundation is starting to crumble and you are becoming more and more out of balance.

In numerous healthy aging studies, researchers have found that a healthy diet, exercise, an engaged mind and high degrees of social belonging seem to be the keys to warding off the signs and symptoms of premature aging. Adding to this body of knowledge are the emerging studies specifically done on the immunomodulating effects of polysaccharides unique to Red Reishi. We are just beginning to catalog the immense benefits gained when these bioactive substances exert their anti-tumor and anti-microbial effects, and their lipid-lowering and glucose-regulating properties.

When taken on a regular basis, Red Reishi essence has profound anti-aging effects. It will help you look and feel more youthful because your body's metabolism will be fine tuned. Due to its glucose lowering and liver enhancing effects, Red Reishi can help you shed those extra pounds you've picked up with age. Since Red Reishi increases the liver's ability to cleanse and detoxify, your skin will be the first to show this new found health. As many individuals will attest, their skin literally glows when taking Red Reishi on a regular basis.

Along with the compliments come more pep and stamina, which will invigorate you and make you feel more physical. As a result, you'll feel more attractive and stronger, and that in turn, can lead to greater satisfaction with life in general.

This incredible mushroom is a true healing force of nature. Red Reishi will help you cope with daily challenges in count-less ways and enjoy a lifetime of optimal wellness, and if you happen to look a little better along the way, so be it!

"I initially started to take Red Reishi for the immune support – I am pleased to report that I not only experienced fewer bouts of illness, my friends have pointed out how fantastic my skin looks! Needless to say, I have made these capsules a regular part of my day!"

Patricia P- mother of four

"Red Reishi has increased and stabilized my energy levels, I have better overall health, acne has been reduced 85%, I feel less stress, emotionally balanced and happy."

Christine S- brand manger

RED
REISHI

Its Role as an Adaptogen

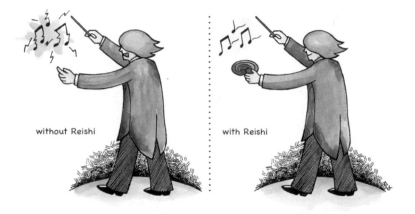

without Reishi   with Reishi

RED REISHI IS WHAT SCIENTISTS CALL AN "ADAPTOGEN". Adaptogens increase the body's general resistance to stress (trauma, anxiety, illness and fatigue), and it does this with few, if any, side effects.

This adaptogenic quality of certain plants is one of nature's great mysteries. The key word being: adapt. Imagine a plant that is able to provide you with the right healing nudge, in the right amount, in the right direction, and at the right time. That is what adaptogens do. Science has not been able to duplicate this confounding yet healing action in any synthetic drug. And true adaptogens are far from common. In fact, only one herb in 300 actually qualifies, and Red Reishi is one of the best among them. A high potency adaptogenic herb, it is known in Traditional Chinese Medicine (TCM) for giving your body what it needs most—the ability to rebound from the unrelenting stress of everyday living. In the process, by helping to rebuild the foundation of healthy longevity, Red Reishi works to balance your body by: enhancing energy levels if you're feeling run down and stagnant and/or, calming you if you're irritable and wired.

The human body continually strives for balance. Anything that moves us away from this natural harmony causes a disruption within our internal systems (or cracks in our foundations), making it more and more difficult for us to experience healthy longevity. So, what we need is something that helps us repair these cracks, and in the process helps our bodies achieve optimal balance again. A good example of this balancing function is the adaptogenic effect that Red Reishi has on blood pressure and cholesterol.

Red Reishi helps to reduce high blood pressure, and yet, because it is an adaptogen, when taken by someone with low blood pressure, the plant offers a gentle boost.

As an adaptogen for cholesterol, Red Reishi will help increase the good (HDL) without raising the bad (LDL) cholesterol counts.

Once again, it's all about balance…

"Being wary of potential side effects, I was looking for a natural alternative to prescription medication to combat my high blood pressure and cholesterol. I decided to try some red reishi capsules and the results blew me away! After only 3 months I had all my levels re-checked and was thrilled with the results, the bad cholesterol (LDL) was noticeably lower. (see lab results below) I am staying on the reishi to maintain my new and improved numbers!"

Arthur O. – retiree

Age: 59 years   Sex: M
Date of Birth: Mar 8 1947
PHN:
Patient's Phone:

Lab No:
Patient ID:
Referring Site ID:

≼xcelleris™
Technologies

Reported by: BC Biomedical Laboratories

Collected on: Feb 24 2007 08:04
Reported on: Feb 24 2007 14:26

Telephone:
Toll Free:
Fax:

Ordered by:
Copy To:

Printed on: 2007-02-26 08:42
Page 1 of 1

Test	Flag	Result	Reference Range
General Chemistry			
Sodium		140	135 -145 mmol/L
Potassium		5	3.5 - 5.0 mmol/L
Urea	H	9.1	2.0 - 9.0 mmol/L
Creatinine	H	139	45 - 110 umol/L
Estimated GFR	L	45	> 59 ml/min/1.73sq.m

Note: eGFR based on serum creatinine, age and gender. This result indicates reduced function, nees further evaluation and follow up: see www.healthservices.gov.bc.ca/msp/protoguides/gps/ckd.pdf

Lipids

	Oct-06	Feb-07		
Cholesterol	6.5	3.9	2.0 - 5.2	mmol/L
		At risk:>6.2 mmol/L		
LDL Cholesterol	4.1	1.8	1.5 - 3.4	mmol/L
		At risk:>3.4 mmol/L		
		An LDL cholesterol level of less than 2.6 mmol/L is suggested for patients with established CAD.		
HDL Cholesterol	1.8	1.7	>0.9	mmol/L
Chol/HDL (Risk Ratio)		2.3	<5.0	
		A ratio of 5.0 in males is associated with average risk. Increased ratios are associated with higher risk for CAD		
Triglycerides	1.4	1.0	<2.3	mmol/L
-Time Since Eating		11.0		h pc

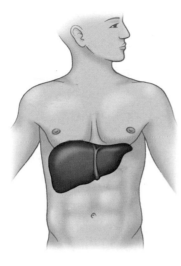

NO ORGAN ENJOYS RED REISHI'S ATTENTION MORE THAN the liver, which is why it is often used by Traditional Chinese Medicine practitioners to aid in the detoxification process. When your liver is happy, everything else is happier... or at least it's all working better. The liver—the largest of the internal organs—is responsible for performing over 500 different chemical functions, some of which include: the metabolism of foods (protein, carbs and fats), the storage of vitamins and minerals, blood sugar control, hormone control, the manufacturing of proteins (including albumin, fibrinogen, and most globulins) and fats (phospholipids, cholesterol), and producing a substance called bile that the body uses for digestion and detoxification.

Environmental poisons, along with an overabundance of food additives, pesticides, herbicides and other horrors, can have your poor liver ready to wave a white flag! It could be working overtime, just barely able to perform the metabolic miracles your body needs. For the average person, consistent support of the liver's detoxification is critical for overall health and longevity, and to maintain a metabolism that is geared towards continual fat loss. In fact, one of the indications of poor liver function may be your body's inability to properly metabolize fat.

"Detoxification is like getting the poisons out of your body, and when you take Red Reishi mushrooms, they assist in getting the liver cleansed out. Reishi helps remove chemicals and other byproducts that are stored in the fat. All of these byproducts that are in the system are basically taking away from energy, so if you remove them you optimize the body's ability to perform more consistently."

Peter S. - two time Olympian and gym owner

Your Liver and Weight Control

Most people understand that the body's metabolism doesn't function properly in those suffering from obesity. According to researchers from Stirling University in Scotland, our exposure to synthetic, organic and inorganic chemicals might be to blame for damaging many of the body's natural weight-control mechanisms, leading to a dysfunctional metabolism and weight gain.

To further support this theory, research published in the International Journal of Obesity indicates that liver toxicity leads to an accumulation of excess body fat, which increases the odds of liver disease and dysfunction. Researchers assessed the liver function of 534 moderately obese (meaning 30-50% over their ideal weight) non-drinkers and found that 24% had abnormal liver enzyme levels and 47% had significant deposits of fat in their livers - a condition called hepatic steatosis, or fatty liver. This study clearly indicates a correlation of moderate obesity with liver dysfunction.

Doctors often assess liver disease or dysfunction by measuring the levels of specific enzymes within the liver. Elevated liver enzymes usually indicate that there is a problem with the liver cells, (*liver function is also measured by other lab tests - PT, PTT, Albumin*) **and many studies show a direct link between excess body fat and these elevated enzyme levels.**

Researchers from the University of Rochester School of Medicine and Dentistry in New York have discovered that elevated liver enzyme concentrations are more frequently found in obese populations than previously thought. Their study indicated that levels of the liver enzyme called ALT (alanine aminotransferase), was elevated in 16 out of 17 obese participants.

The good news is that researchers have proven that liver function can be corrected once a person loses a significant portion of body fat. In one study, patients who lost 54% of their excess body weight by following a specialized high protein diet showed considerable improvement in their liver function. These findings confirm what was discussed in the earlier research cited.

Japanese researchers have also discovered that excess body fat is linked with liver disorders. Research from 1,591 people over a 10-year period, indicated that obesity is more closely related to liver dysfunction than to any other abnormalities.

There's no doubt that one of the keys to effective weight loss and to good health and longevity is to keep the liver healthy and functioning optimally. Taking a Red Reishi supplement on a daily basis can play a significant role in your body's detoxification process…but that's just part of the story. Preliminary studies also show that Red Reishi extract is an effective aid in serious liver disorders like hepatitis B by helping to reduce elevated liver enzymes - an indication of the repair of damaged liver cells.

When you read something like this, you can see why Red Reishi is one very important mushroom! It helps to reduce the wear and tear on your body's organs, and tissues; and increase your resistance to infections, such as viruses, bacteria, fungus and external toxins, and enhance the support of your body's immune and nervous system, all the while working to maintain a healthy metabolism that promotes healthy fat loss, increased energy, concentration, mood, sleep, and a general sense of well-being. It almost seems too good to be true! But as you'll soon find out, Red Reishi is not called the "Real Magic Mushroom™" for nothing.

Red Reishi is Nature's crowning achievement in adaptogen science. Herbalists use Red Reishi to support allergies, bronchitis, viral infections and hypertension. Its adaptogenic effect also extends to enhance detoxification, improve mood and appetite, vigor, and mental alertness.

CHAPTER TWO

THE "S" WORD

Battle Stress

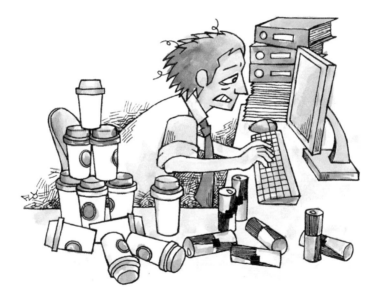

Besides detoxification, stress reduction is a key feature of Red Reishi's adaptogenic heroism. We know that no one escapes the stress of today's busy world. We're fighting noise, pollution, overwork, bad diets, and more. The constant battle creates a powerful - and what's worse, *continuous* level of stress and distress. This comes with a huge cost – bad health.

There has been a lot of research done on the effect of stress, with at least one researcher - Kenneth Pelletier (Stanford Trained Alternative and Integrative Medicine Expert) - coming to the conclusion that in America, between 80 and 90 percent of all illness is linked to stress; 75 to 90 percent of all visits to the doctor are for stress and anxiety-related conditions!

Our body reacts to stress – and the system really can't tell the difference between an attacking tiger and somebody that cuts you off in traffic – by producing two powerful chemicals. They are the hormones Epinephrine (Adrenalin) and Cortisol, which are often referred to as the "fight or flight" hormones. These are produced by the adrenal glands; two triangular shaped glands that sit beside your kidneys; Adrenalin for short-term stress, and Cortisol for long-term stress.

These hormones are "designed" to get us ready to either fight whatever it is that's causing our stress (tiger, traffic, taxes), or run away (flight) – not usually an option any more, especially with regard to taxes... To do this, Adrenalin increases the heart rate, raises blood sugar levels, and diverts blood to the most important organs, driving your body way out of balance. This reaction has been honed through centuries of evolution to help us to survive in a dangerous world. However, it was originally "designed" to work only for very short periods of time – just long enough to win the fight or escape from the tiger.

> *"At first I thought, "Well what can a mushroom do?" But I was amazed at the extra energy Reishi gives you...this is my new secret weapon!"*
>
> Kid C. - popular morning show radio host

"I have noticed the benefits of Reishi by way of increased energy, focus and endurance – without the worry of an energy crash or sleepless nights that come with energy drinks or tablets. I recommend this product to anyone who wants to excel in sports or just wants to feel energized and at the top of their game."

John C. - former NHL player

Stress and Immunity

One of the effects of both Epinephrine (Adrenalin) and Cortisol is to temporarily suppress parts of the immune system. This effect is so powerful that Adrenalin is used in emergencies to treat patients having a life-threatening allergic reaction - to nuts, for example – which is basically the result of your immune system going into overdrive against a substance that the body sees as "foreign". Chronically elevated levels of Adrenalin and Cortisol will certainly have an effect on one's immune system, leading to all kinds of infections.

Imagine what this suppression does to your health if you are constantly under stress.

> *"I have a high pressure job and it often takes quite a toll on my nerves. A co-worker suggested trying a Reishi essence supplement. I was amazed at how fast it worked... within one week I felt substantially less stressed out and also noticed my energy levels improved. I feel better than I have in years."*
>
> **Brian C. - stock promoter**

Nowadays we are bathed in stress of one kind or another almost continually. Our system is "on" way more than its designer(s) intended, continually chipping away at our foundation and destroying our balance.

One of the big problems with this is that Cortisol, which is slower to react than Adrenaline, ends up hanging around a lot longer – even after the stress has gone. This can cause a whole host of problems like: obesity, depression, Fibromyalgia, immune suppression (constantly getting sick and taking a long time to recover), loss of libido, poor digestion, excess inflammation (think; my aching back), allergies, loss of muscle and bone (wasting syndrome and osteoporosis), skin disorders (Eczema, Psoriasis, Acne, etc.) The list goes on...

Getting Older and Fatter Through Age

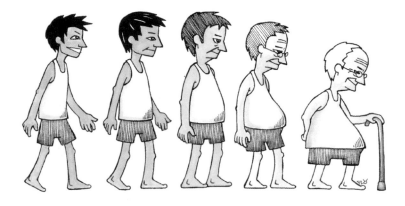

Almost anyone would agree that chronic stress ages people. The fact is that, until recently, scientists studying aging could only theorize as to why. We are now coming to understand that the majority of our cells have a finite number of times they are able to divide. Our body's repair system depends on cell division, but it seems that every time cells divide, they lose a small piece of DNA called a "telomere". It is believed that the shortening of these telomeres is, to a significant degree, responsible for the aging process. In 2004, researchers from the University of California discovered that women who had the highest levels of perceived stress have telomeres that are much shorter than women who experience low stress. The researchers concluded that these shortened telomeres were equivalent to at least one decade of additional aging.

Another effect of stress on aging is from our old friend Cortisol. Cortisol is one of the biggest culprits. It is known to eat away at our foundation by degrading muscle tissue (the metabolic engine of the body) and, according to research published in the Journal of the American Geriatrics Society, loss of lean body mass (i.e. muscle) is the number one reason we age prematurely.

Cortisol can also be blamed on our inability to lose fat as we age. Nasty stuff. In fact, the longer your stress response is turned "on", the more body fat you accumulate—especially in the abdominal cavity. By the way, abdominal fat is also the most dangerous form of fat your body carries, due to the fact that it impacts the major organs and can easily increase your susceptibility to heart disease and diabetes. Cortisol can also lead to unhealthy weight gain by affecting the degree to which you crave certain foods. Constant stress can easily deplete levels of a "feel-good" chemical in the body called Serotonin. Research shows us that when Serotonin levels are low, or when they are unable to remain in their special pockets called synaptic junctions, a condition called "Emotional Eating" results and chronic cravings for sweet and starchy foods (yes, the very foods responsible for easy fat storage) become next to impossible to ignore. After all, we don't call these types of foods "comfort foods" for nothing.

One of the main reasons that we experience emotional eating is that chronic stress reduces the levels of the amino acid Tryptophan, which is essential to the manufacture of Serotonin in our bodies. Stress can deplete Tryptophan levels by up to 90 percent in extreme situations,

leaving very little for production of the Serotonin that helps us control our cravings. Incidentally, low levels of Serotonin may also lead to depression – it goes without saying how important a proper balance is for a healthy state of mind!

"I had been suffering from stress induced headaches and hormonal imbalance and nothing I had been trying worked. I finally tried a Japanese grown Reishi product and it was a profound experience – it rejuvenated my body; and gave me balance and clarity."

Ashie H- charity organizer

"My skin looks healthier and younger, people have been saying I am looking so well. Another great benefit is it has lifted the depression I've had for a very long time. People have also commented that I seem happier now. My life situation has not changed at all, it's just that I don't get upset like I used to. I have just an overall healthier feeling and I'm sure there are other good things going on in my body that I'm not yet aware of."

Olive P- R.N.

People use many effective de-stressing strategies from meditation and exercise, to petting an animal, or switching to a natural whole foods diet. But they can still use extra help. Thankfully, unique elements in Red Reishi act as building blocks of chemicals that are important to proper functioning of our nerves, and hormonal system, and adjusts the effects of these chemicals as needed; the very definition of an adaptogen. Red Reishi can give you back your balance.

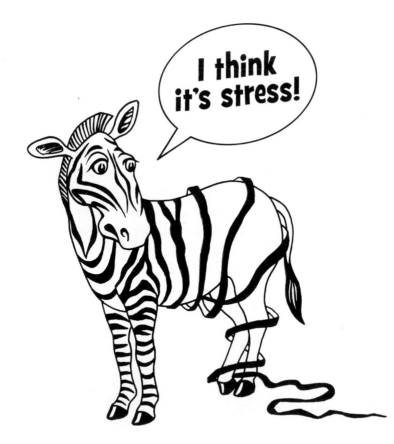

The Quest for Energy

If you're like most people, you share the number one minor health complaint: you want more energy. You'd like to feel pep in the morning, and stamina and alertness to get through your busy day. And it doesn't stop there – you'd also like a good measure of sustained energy to enjoy activities late into the evening.

Perhaps more than anything, the Red Reishi mushroom is valued as a tonic that supplies a steady flow of energy that you can count on day after day. When you start taking Red Reishi, you'll usually notice the energy boost before any other benefit. The energy from Red Reishi is not the hyped-up frenzy from a caffeinated drink. Instead, Reishi's energy arrives smooth and steady as a new vitality that will surprise you with its reliability.

This is one of the primary reasons Red Reishi was so revered by the ancient Oriental herbalists. They secretly shared with royal dynasties the benefits of how the prize mushroom worked directly on the life energy or "Qi" (pronounced chee). Reishi and Qi are sublime partners. The way Reishi enhances this all-pervasive vital energy is not fully mapped out yet, but its evidence is undeniable due to thousands of years of human usage.

In the West, doctors regard energy as a simple biochemical equation: nutrients and oxygen into the cells produce ATP or units of energy used in thousands of biochemical processes. That equation takes place in the Kreb's cycle of the cell's mitochondria.

In the East, the traditional view of how energy is cultivated and enhanced follows the amazing path of physical and universal Qi, which can be gathered from nature as well as strengthened within the human body. There are many types of Qi in the body: wei qi, ying qi, yuan qi and zong qi. Acupuncture is the insertion of needles at various points on the body to regulate the flow and distribution of vital energy. Red Reishi enhances this energy (without the use of needles!) and makes you feel great at the same time.

Today modern medicine is in all parts of the world and doctors in both East and West share the same biochemical view of cellular energy production. However, the emergence of integrative medicine is a new field that blends the best of traditional healing systems from around the world with the scientific foundation of modern medicine. As more researchers confirm the validity of Traditional Chinese Medicine herbal remedies such as the Red Reishi mushroom, the respect for what the ancient herbalists knew grows profound.

"Like most men in their 40s, my life had slowed down. With less and less sports taking up what little spare time I had, to no surprise the kilos started creeping onto my midsection. Having been a triathlete in my late 20s and early 30s, I started a workout plan with lots of variety. However, I found it was harder and harder to maintain the workout plan as I simply no longer had the energy that I had had when I was younger. So after a bit of on-line research I made the trip

to the health food store and purchased some Red Reishi.

The effects were, to say the least, surprising if not shocking. Within three days I had gone from 10 large cups of coffee a day to one. In my entire adult life I have had an energy "dead zone" from 1pm to 3pm: it was now gone. Not only did I now have the energy to stick to my new workout program, I now had the energy again to go out socializing after work and not be exhausted the next morning. More importantly, I am out there trying new things again. All this on only one capsule a day.

So now, four months later and having stuck to my workout program and little diet rules like no carbs after 7 pm, I am now almost 50 lbs lighter. I now have an excuse to buy a whole new wardrobe, and am outlasting players in their 20s on my beach volleyball team. The Reishi Essence capsules on their own did not get me there, but as part of an overall exercise and diet program, they played an essential part. Without them, I do not believe I would have enjoyed the success I had over the last four months. It is a great feeling, being able to sit here in loose-fitting jeans with a waist of 32 when back in January I was a very tight fit in a 36 waist."

Peter A.- communications manager

CHAPTER THREE

MAINTAINING IMMUNITY AS WE AGE

WHEN WE ARE YOUNG WE CAN HAVE BOUTS OF ILLNESS like colds and flu from time to time, but we usually bounce back quickly — and, many times, stronger than before. Youth is synonymous with a robust immune system; one that is able to handle most viruses, bacteria, fungi, parasites and almost anything else that can be thrown at it. Unfortunately as we get older, our immunity is often not nearly as strong as it was in youth, which is why common viral infections like colds and the flu can quickly turn into dangerous and even fatal complications like pneumonia. In fact, upper respiratory problems become such an issue with advanced age that over 61,000 people die from these conditions each year alone.

To help you to understand how it is that Red Reishi can be so effective at strengthening our immune system, it's helpful to know a little more about how the system works. In fact, it's like a fascinating little army, with many soldiers – each having their own specialized function – battlefields, and tactical weapons.

Warriors en guarde!

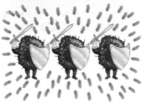

Our immune system protects us when some sort of damage, or infection, occurs. The system is very complex and made up of an army of different types of cells in the blood stream that come to our defense when an intruder is detected. It is very important to our well-being that this system be ready to "march into battle" at all times. The army analogy actually works very well, because the fight against invaders such as bacteria, viruses, and cancer cells is tough, trench warfare.

The immune system is made up of a number of cells, tissues and organs that work together and have various jobs. They destroy invading bacteria and viruses, consume dead cell material, secrete chemicals to recruit other cells to the fight against infection, cause inflammation, and do other very important work to keep us healthy. It's an amazing, complicated system that, if nourished, works hard in the background to defend us against disease. The miracle of immunity is we never even know it's there! It's almost like having an invisible bodyguard on call—24 hours a day.

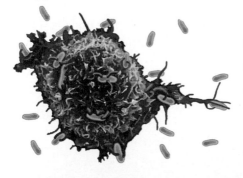

The problem is that we tend to lose much of our defense system as we age. Both the numbers of specialized immune warriors and their ability to react to danger decline as we get older. This is where specialized nutrients that are found in the plant kingdom—and as you will see, in exceptional quantities within Red Reishi—come to the aid of our immune system. Some of these nutrients are even able to "turn on" or "activate" the most powerful warriors our immune system contains. Once these immune cells are activated, watch out! The end result is the annihilation of almost anything the body perceives as a threat to our health.

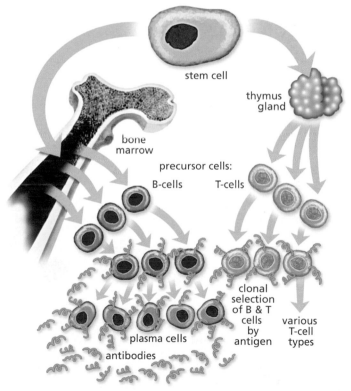

stem cell

thymus gland

bone marrow

precursor cells:

B-cells   T-cells

clonal selection of B & T cells by antigen

various T-cell types

plasma cells

antibodies

The cells of the immune system all originate from "stem cells" which are produced in bone marrow. Stem cells develop into various different kinds of white blood cells, depending on what's needed to respond to invasion (e.g. infection, bacterial, viral, etc.). Our immune system has the remarkable ability to tell the difference between the cells which belong to our body, and those "foreign" cells which do not. Once a foreign cell is detected, the system is mobilized and launches an attack against it, be it a virus, bacteria, or whatever it is that triggered the response.

Here are some of the many soldiers that can be recruited:

WHITE BLOOD CELLS

Also called leucocytes, these are the cells in the body that defend us against infectious diseases, and foreign bodies. White blood cells are crucial to the body's defense against infections. There are a great variety of types, divided into classes based on whether or not they contain granules, which are packages of enzymes – bombs, if you will – that can be used to destroy invaders.

GRANULOCYTES:

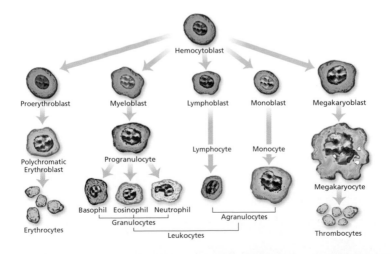

These cells contain packages, or granules, of enzymes and other chemicals that are released to digest invading viruses or bacteria.

- Basophils – Basophils are white blood cells that release Histamines. Histamines cause blood vessels to become "leaky" in the area of infection, allowing other immune system components to flood the site. This leakage causes the swelling and redness in an injury.

- Eosinophils – Primarily deal with infections by parasites. They contain several kinds of enzymes that are toxic to both parasite and host tissues.

- Neutrophils – Neutrophils deal with defense against bacterial or fungal infection and other very small inflammatory processes, and are usually first responders to microbial infection; their work, and death in large numbers, forms pus.

- Agranulocytes – These white blood cells do not contain granules, and function in a different way.

- Mast cells – Similar to the neutrophil, it is found in the lungs, skin, tongue, and linings of the nose and intestine. They are responsible for the symptoms of allergy. Mast cells release Heparin (which prevents blood clots), and Histamine into a wound site.

- Lymphocytes –The blood has three types of lymphocytes:
    1. B cells: B cells make chemicals called antibodies that bind to invading bacteria or viruses either to modify them so they don't work anymore, or identify them

to the immune system for destruction. B cells not only make antibodies that bind to invaders, but after an attack, some B cells will retain the ability to produce an antibody to serve as a 'memory' system, allowing a faster response the next time the bacterium or virus gets into our body.

2. T cells: T cells co-ordinate the immune response and are important in the defense against bacteria that have invaded cells. Some T cells are able to kill virus-infected and tumorous cells, others produce chemicals, called cytokines, which regulate, or "help" the immune system.

3. Natural Killer cells: As their name implies, Natural Killer (NK) cells are able to eliminate cells of the body which are displaying a signal to kill them, because they have been infected by a virus, or have become cancerous.

MACROPHAGES:

Their name comes from the Greek word meaning "big eater" (makros=large, phagein=eat), and macrophages are an important part of our immune system. Their role is to engulf and digest cellular debris and infectious agents ("pathogens"), and to stimulate other immune cells to respond to the infection. Remember the computer game "Pac-Man"? That little guy that gobbled up everything in his path? That's what macrophages are like.

Macrophages originate from specific white blood cells called monocytes. Monocytes are attracted to a damaged site by a range of chemicals either produced when a cell dies, or chemicals released by mast cells, basophils, or other macrophages already at the site of the infection. Polysaccharides (found in the highest quantity in Japanese Red Reishi) – primarily beta-glucan – are known for their incredible ability to help macrophages communicate with other immune cells, and to activate the macrophages in order for them to effectively neutralize or "gobble up" the invaders.

As you can see from this short list of just a few members of the immune system army, it is very complex, with a lot of intertwined functions. It's important that it be working as well as it can. Taking Japanese Red Reishi can help.

"I had been suffering with depression and low energy that was getting slowly worse, and irritable bowel syndrome (IBS) certainly didn't help matters. I am always traveling around for work and this can really run you down, so I was not coping very well with it. A trusted friend in the health industry recommended that I try a Reishi mushroom supplement; within one month my body and energy was completely changed. At first I just thought I was having a good day or a good week, but I soon realized that this change was permanent! My IBS symptoms are truly all but gone, my mood is upbeat and I just feel so much more vital than I did before. I've got my partner on Red Reishi now, and I would wholeheartedly recommend it. It has had a drastically positive impact on my life."

Sean T. - interior designer

A Key to Successful Aging

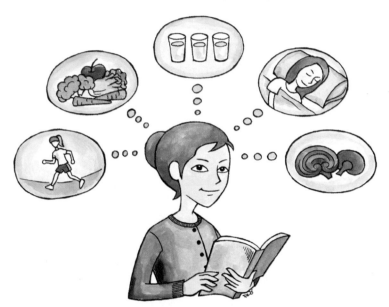

AGING IS NOT ALWAYS ACCOMPANIED BY ILLNESS, BUT getting older does come with an increased risk of many diseases, disorders, and dysfunctions. Elderly people do have a higher rate of chronic health problems: lung problems, hardening of the arteries, infections, auto-immune disorders, and cancer. Often these problems don't show themselves until they've been with us for many years; they sneak up on us.

Our immune system protects against diseases, viruses,

bacteria, fungi, and cancerous cells. When we are young, our immune system is in full operation; it destroys the bad guys – the viruses, the unhealthy cells, the infections etc. before they can destroy us. But our immune system changes as we age, and not for the better…

Changes to Our Immune System as We Age

For a good example of how our immune system changes as we age, let's take a look at the gland called the Thymus. The Thymus is the site where T cells mature, and is one of the major organs of the immune system. It begins to shrink after adolescence (some studies indicate that it starts to shrink as soon as we're born), and by middle age it is only about 15% of its maximum size.

Some T cells directly kill foreign particles, while some help coordinate other parts of the immune system which are specialized to attack different types of infection. The bottom line is that they are very important, and any reduction in the number or quality of T cells can have a major impact on our well-being. Unfortunately, as we age, the number of T cells along with their ability to divide and form new T cells, declines. Researchers from David Geffen School of Medicine at UCLA have even discovered that many of these T cells can actually turn against us in advanced age, further reducing our ability to defend against incoming invaders. This causes a weakening of the parts of the immune system controlled by these cells. There has been a demonstrated increase in risk of death in individuals with low numbers of T cells.

In general, there is a slow, steady decrease in the strength of our immune system after young adulthood. In addition to the reduction in T cell number and function, B cells (which produce antibodies) don't work as well, and there are fewer of them. When the body is exposed to bacteria or other micro-organisms—by exposure or by immunization—fewer protective antibodies may be formed of a lower quality, or formed at a slower rate.

While it's true that everyone shows a decline in immune function with age, it's also coming to light that stress can make things worse, by aging our immune system faster. We'll talk about T cells in a moment, but first, the SECRET WEAPON.

Japanese Red Reishi

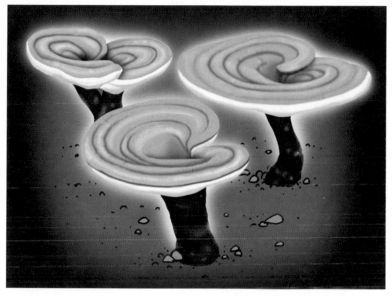

RESEARCH HAS SHOWN THAT JAPANESE RED REISHI can bring reinforcements to your body's immunity army. It strengthens the body's immune system and helps it to maintain a strong immune response as we age.

Just like you can't expect an army to go into battle without food, water, and weapons, you can't expect your immune system to work well on a daily basis without the support that it needs. Japanese Red Reishi mushrooms are very complex and contain many substances that contribute to its medicinal qualities. For example, one of the substances found in Red Reishi (the highest amounts of which are found in the Japanese variety) is the Polysaccharide—a molecule made of many sugar molecules linked together—called Beta-glucan, and it happens to be one of the most exciting immune enhancing substances ever discovered.

Beta-glucans have the unique ability to aid in the communication between major parts of our immune system, helping them to respond more quickly to infection. Remember earlier when we talked about our Pac-Men (our macrophages) gobbling up the bad stuff? These polysaccharides within Red Reishi help to "talk" to them, to communicate that they'd better get a move on and fight off the bad guys. Other mushrooms may contain Polysaccharides, but not nearly in the concentration found in properly cultivated and processed Japanese Red Reishi. Japanese Red Reishi is believed to be one of the most powerful allies our immune system could ever have!

"Since I started taking Japanese Red Reishi, I noticed I had no hayfever this past spring, no colds and managed to avoid getting the FLU that my roommate had. I still felt great-- despite the fact that I was working very hard and under a lot of stress."

Michelle M.- sales executive

More on Japanese Red Reishi's Magnificent Beta-Glucans

Beta-glucans, found in Japanese Red Reishi, are such an important part of our whole disease-fighting machine that we want to spend a few more moments talking about them. Let's start with the flu. We've all had it (actually there are many different varieties of flu virus, but all of them pretty much feel the same—lousy). We don't want it. The good news is that researchers have proven that Beta-glucan is effective in fighting the influenza virus. According to the U.S. Center for Disease Control and Prevention, a combination of flu and pneumonia is the fifth highest killer of adults 65 and over. The flu hits us much harder as we age, due to our weakened immune systems. It accounts for nearly 60,000 deaths every year.

Beta-glucan sounds like good news...but what else can it do? Researchers from Kobe Pharmaceutical University, Japan, have explored the effect of Beta-glucans on T cell activity. They studied the anti-tumor functions of Beta-glucan and found that it was extremely effective at enhancing cellular immunity.

Researchers also found that Beta-glucan increased production of Interferon gamma and Interleukin—two powerful weapons the immune system uses to battle invaders. Another study investigated what happened when Beta-glucan was given to mice infected with bacteria that cause a disease called listeriosis. Listeriosis occurs in newborns, elderly patients, and patients whose immune system is damaged in some way, for example, those with HIV. Those not treated with Beta-glucan died within three days of inoculation with the listeriosis bacteria. But, the survival rate of mice treated with Beta-glucan was 60 percent on the 10th day. The researchers reported significant increases in T cell activity in the spleen; with macrophages producing over two times as much Interleukin.

Aside from all of the wonderful immune supporting actions discovered for polysaccharides like Beta-glucan—especially their effect on communication between cells, Red Reishi also contains a protein that stimulates the production of monocytes and T cells, some of the most important members of our internal army. In fact there are over TWO HUNDRED different substances in Red Reishi, and they all work together in marvelous synergy to help make your immune system the best that it can be. Once again, it is the Japanese variety of Red Reishi that offers the highest levels of these life enhancing compounds.

Basic Training for Your Immune System

The effect of adding Japanese Red Reishi to your daily schedule is like training the heart and lungs through aerobic exercise, or training the muscles by lifting weights. Japanese Red Reishi actually trains the body's immune system and nervous system to perform better. Natural medicine experts are beginning to suspect that the body's immune system needs this training.

We're born with an immature system, a system that requires training through childhood fevers and early combats with infections such as chickenpox and stomach flu. Long-term studies have shown that children who live in challenging environments have a higher success rate defeating certain cancers. Their immune systems took on early struggles with dirt, poverty, filth, and bugs, and grew robust as a result. That's why it's so important to just let kids be kids. We're not suggesting a daily helping of dirt, but we do know that a daily dose of Japanese Red Reishi can provide that training ground for your immune system—at any age.

Japanese Red Reishi can be taken daily, without any side effects to help boost the power of your own immune system and to help manage powerful stress hormones such as Cortisol and Norepinephrine, and a wide range of other compounds such as enzymes, neurotransmitters, catecholamines, and prostaglandins.

Many of the other components of Red Reishi have been studied and proven to have positive effects on blood pressure and cholesterol levels, improved immunity, and general health.

> *"Since I started taking Japanese Red Reishi, I'm more focused and can bounce back faster from jetlag. Although I still have the same amount of stress in my life, I feel that my response to it is much stronger, and my immunity doesn't suffer like it used to, from getting run down."*
>
> Marcello L. -couture fashion boutique owner

The Immune System
AND RED REISHI

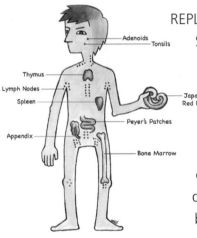

Adenoids
Tonsils
Thymus
Lymph Nodes
Spleen
Japanese Red Reishi
Peyer's Patches
Appendix
Bone Marrow

EVERY DAY, YOUR BODY REPLACES HUNDREDS OF THOU-SANDS of cells that are either old – in cell terms – or damaged in some way. Many things can damage cells: elevated stress chemicals (i.e. Cortisol), chemical pollution, sun damage, mechanical injury, bad diet, etc. Dead or damaged cells must be replaced for the body to keep working. Replacement cells are produced by a process that involves the splitting or dividing of one cell to form two new ones. Those two cells split to form four, then those four split to form eight, and so on. If we are able to produce healthy versions of our old cells, we retain youthfulness, but, when these new cells are inferior to the old ones, aging makes its biggest impact.

Cells contain genes, which are the chemical instructions that tell a cell how to grow, and what to do (become a hair cell, a liver cell, a muscle cell, or whatever its destiny). These genes are kind of like blueprints for a new house, without the blue-prints, the house doesn't get built—at least not the way it was originally intended to!

Each time a cell divides, this gene material, called DNA, must make a perfect copy of itself to pass on to the new cell that will result from the division. In the vast majority of cases, this duplication of DNA is performed flawlessly, however, in a small percentage of cases, mistakes are made in the copying process, and a change is made to the DNA (the blueprint is a little damaged or parts of it are no longer legible). This change is called a "mutation", or a "deletion", because it results in a change to the cell's instructions. A mutation (or deletion) can drastically affect how the cell works (kind of like building a house with a blurred copy of the plans).

If a mutation occurs in the genes that control growth, the cell will become a cancer cell, undergo uncontrolled division, and form a tumor. When normal cells change, or mutate, into cancer cells, some of their characteristics change, and they can be recognized by our immune system as damaged and identified as "foreign" (no longer welcome). These foreign cells will be attacked by our immune system, and eliminated. Tumors develop when our immune system breaks down, or isn't strong enough to repel the invaders and is overwhelmed.

Again we say that it is vital that our immune system be as strong and healthy as possible, so that we can fight off the damage that is done to our cells on a daily basis. Regular consumption of Japanese Red Reishi has been shown to stimulate the production of Interferon, and Interleukins I and II, potent natural anti-cancer substances produced in our body. Furthermore, researchers claim that polysaccharides—especially Beta-glucans—have been shown to possess powerful anti-tumor properties. Japanese Red Reishi can help to combat cancer in a couple of ways:

1) RED REISHI STIMULATES THE PRODUCTION OF INTERFERON

Reishi has been shown to stimulate the production of Interferon. Interferon is a protein—actually a group of proteins—produced by the immune system, that slow down the growth of viruses. They also activate macrophages and natural killer (NK) cells, which destroy invading bacteria, viruses, and cancer cells.

2) RED REISHI STIMULATES THE PRODUCTION OF INTERLEUKIN 1 AND 2

Interleukins are a group of chemicals (33 different types) that function in communication, or signaling, between cells of the immune system. They have many functions, including promoting and activating killer cells, stimulation of antibody production, stimulation of blood cell growth, and stimulating different types of interferon production.

A major effect of Reishi on cancer cells happens through its effect on the class of White Blood cells called T-lymphocytes, so we'll look at them in more detail next. This next section is going to get quite technical, but we think it's important to have this kind of information to help you understand why Japanese Red Reishi is so effective.

Diabetes

Diabetes is a disorder that results in a higher than normal level of blood sugar in the body. There are two types of diabetes. Type I is due to a lack of insulin production, which is a hormone secreted by the pancreas. The function of this hormone is to regulate blood sugar.

Most people with diabetes have the Type II variety (associated with hyper-insulinemia and insulin resistance). This form of diabetes is more commonly related to obesity, poor nutrition, and lack of exercise. The primary treatment for both types is insulin injections, or oral medications; both of which have side effects. The possible blood sugar lowering effect of a component of Red Reishi, polysaccharides known as ganoderans, has been investigated in several studies. One such study concluded, "the administration of (Reishi extract) to normal mice elicited a hypoglycemic effect (caused a decrease in the blood sugar level)." This effect may be used to treat patients who are borderline Type II diabetes.

Obesity—the Diabetes Connection

Type II diabetes—representing over 90% of all diabetic cases, occurs when insulin-receptor sites on the cells become resistant, or insensitive to the hormone. When this happens, insulin can't bind and move blood sugar into the cells, and both blood sugar and blood-insulin levels remain elevated.

The fact remains that well over 80 percent of Type II diabetics

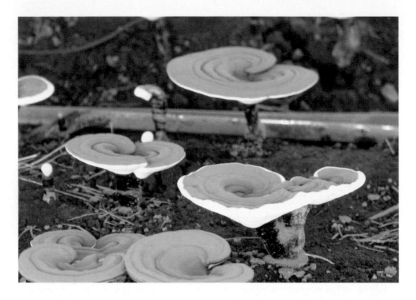

are also obese. Diabesity is a commonly used expression that infers a strong correlation between excess body fat and Type II diabetes. Researchers have known about this for many years, but they have never been able to pinpoint the exact mechanism by which this condition occurs. There are many theories linking the cause of Type II diabetes to obesity, but only a few have been scientifically validated.

Any health practitioner will tell you that the best way to avoid fully blown diabetes is by losing excess body fat. Losing excess fat enhances insulin sensitivity within the cells of the body – in turn, reducing the body's need to over-produce insulin (hyper-insulinemia).

In January of 2001, researchers from the University of Pennsylvania School of Medicine in Philadelphia announced the discovery of a new peptide believed to be the hidden link between Type II diabetes and obesity. The peptide, resistin (for resistance to insulin)—produced by the body's fat cells—was shown to impair blood sugar control and insulin action when given to healthy mice. When resistin was inhibited in obese mice, it regulated blood sugar control and enhanced insulin action (resistin levels are greatly elevated in obesity).

Over the last few years, researchers have found that the overall amount of fat we carry is not nearly as important as where the majority of that fat is located. The amount of fat we carry in our abdominal region appears to play a pivotal role in the development of Type II diabetes. The discovery that increased resistin levels were found in human abdominal fat cells appeared in the prestigious journal, Lancet, in January 2002. This could explain the increased risk of Type II diabetes in abdominally obese people.

Even though nearly one million people are diagnosed with diabetes each year, millions more may be unaware that they are living with this devastating condition. The good news is, research shows that we can, at the very least, eliminate our chances of ever coming face-to-face with this destructive disease by lowering our excess blood sugar levels through exercise, proper diet and now, with the amazing Japanese Red Reishi.

Anti-inflammatory Effects

Many researchers have found that Reishi is a potent anti-inflammatory agent. Extracts of the fruiting body (the part of the plant above the surface of the soil) worked both when taken internally, or applied to the skin. The active compound was isolated, identified and found to be equivalent in anti-inflammatory activity to hydrocortisone. The good news is that it doesn't have the typical side effects associated with steroids or non-steroidal anti-inflammatory drugs (NSAIDs) such as aspirin, Ibuprofen, or Naprosyn. One of the major side-effects associated with NSAIDs is damage to the stomach lining, which can eventually lead to excessive bleeding. Chronic use of NSAIDs can lead to kidney and liver damage.

Japanese Red Reishi can help to reduce symptoms of allergies, and its anti-inflammatory activity has potential applications in preventing the development of such diverse diseases as mental decline, Alzheimer's disease, intestinal disorders, diabetes, cardiovascular disease and arthritis.

"When I was first diagnosed with rheumatoid arthritis, my son was not even two years old... I was given a really bleak outlook on the illness... they flat out said that this is a destructive illness and in 2 years you will stop working. In 5 years you will be in a wheelchair, and if we don't treat this, you are on your way to that wheelchair right now. I decided to research a new natural medicine and I did as much as I could as quickly as I

could. I had to just really search inside myself to see what was going to work for me. What was going to keep my son's mom walking ... So I took the western medicine for years and years and at the same time I would balance it with supplements and powerful super foods. When I included the Japanese Red Reishi the very first time, I took it on a day that I was taking a very serious prescription drug. When it got to the end of the day I realized that I didn't sleep all day; that I actually got up and could go outside. I definitely was feeling stronger and feeling more like myself. I think the significant difference that I feel when I'm taking Japanese Red Reishi on a med day is that I can be balanced and feeling better and I can go about my regular activities. On a good day when I am feeling fantastic, the good work that the Reishi is doing just makes me stronger."

Honnor M.- Interior Designer

Cardiovascular Benefits

HELP WITH HYPERTENSION AND HIGH CHOLESTEROL

Japanese Red Reishi can help and treat another top killer: cardiovascular disease. The protection Japanese Red Reishi offers against heart disease and stroke is truly remarkable because it can lower many different risk factors. This is due to its high content of heart-saving substances like sterols,

ganoderic acids (Reishi is the only known source of this unique phytonutrient), coumarin, mannitol and polysaccharides. For example, researchers in China found that Red Reishi improved the blood flow and lowered oxygen consumption in heart muscle. And in a six-month clinical trial performed in a university hospital in Tokyo, nearly half (47.5%) of 53 hypertensive patients lowered their blood pressure by 10-19 mmHg, and 10% of the subjects dropped their pressures 20-29 mmHg (both systolic and diastolic readings) after taking Japanese Red Reishi extract. Similar results were seen in a Chinese clinical trial, without any side effects.

Experts believe that the **ganoderic acids**, in particular, lower triglyceride levels, lower cholesterol, lower blood pressure, reduce platelet stickiness (to prevent clotting) and even help correct irregular heart beats. In fact, in 54 patients with hypertension that did not respond to conventional medication, taking Red Reishi extract three times a day for four weeks was enough to lower blood pressure significantly, according to a study reported by Burton Goldberg in his best selling book, Heart Disease.   One can only imagine how the incidence of cardiovascular disease will be reduced when Japanese Red Reishi catches on in the Western hemisphere.

Healthy Aging and Vitality

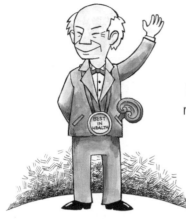

The ancient Chinese believed that Red Reishi is useful for enhancing vital energy, increasing brain function and preventing forgetfulness. It can refresh the body and mind, delay aging and help us to enjoy a long life. The importance of retaining memory into old age could be related to the Taoist belief that sickness was caused by past misconducts and that the patient had to remember the misconducts, record them and then destroy the record. This belief placed a strong emphasis on memory in the maintenance of health and longevity.

Recent reports from the United States indicate that inflammation plays a central role in the development of a variety of diseases such as Alzheimer's and cardiovascular disease. This research has the propensity of linking the historical uses of Reishi in promoting longevity, with current Western scientific theory. The interesting connections are: (1) Reishi has been used for thousands of years to prevent memory loss in old age; (2) Reishi has anti-inflammatory properties; (3) There is a component of inflammation that is involved in the development of Alzheimer's disease; and (4) Alzheimer's disease appears to be improved in patients who take anti-inflammatories on a regular basis.

Research in mice found Red Reishi to be an excellent anti-inflammatory agent. The water extract of the fruiting body was effective when swallowed, against two types of inflammation; carrageenan-induced acute and formalin-induced chronic inflammatory paw edema. A different extract was active as an anti-inflammatory agent both by mouth and when rubbed on the skin. The active compound was found to be equivalent in anti-inflammatory activity to hydrocortisone, a steroid—with none of the side effects.

Immune Support

As we've mentioned earlier, some of the compounds found in Japanese Red Reishi mushrooms—primarily polysaccharides—have been shown to boost our immune system.

A paper reported the results of a clinical trial conducted between August 2000 and April 2001 at the People's Hospital of Lishui City, Zhejiang Province, People's Republic of China. One conclusion was the mixed polysaccharides have an apparent role in controlling and improving the immunity. After taking Reishi, nonspecific immunity of the body is enhanced, improvements in the secretion of IgA (an antibody that protects against infections of the mucous membranes lining the mouth, airways, and digestive tract), increase in the function of monocytes, macrophages and in the activity of NK cells, and in keeping the immunological balance and stability of the body.

Cancer Support

The same study (referred to above), examined the effectiveness of mushroom polysaccharides as an adjunct therapy to improve the immune function of cancer patients undergoing other therapies. They concluded, among other things that:

Polysaccharides can inhibit the production of cancer cells, change the physiological condition of cancer cells, inhibit the growth and transference of cancer cells, relieve the poisoning action of the anti-cancer drugs, improve the patients sleep and appetite and result in overall improvement of the symptoms.

Polysaccharides counteract the complications caused by chemotherapy and radiation, which includes white blood cell reduction. They play an excellent helper role as an adjunct for treatment. In many cases, cancer patients don't die from the actual cancer, but from the complications of treatment - immune suppression and its subsequent infections.

Dr. Ito of Japan discovered the positive effect of Reishi in preventing the spread of cancer in laboratory mice. The Japanese Cancer Society also released their research data on the effectiveness of Reishi against sarcoma 180. Research on the relationship between Reishi and cancer is just beginning and more tests are being conducted; but Reishi is recognized for playing a role in preventing spontaneous death in cancer patients.

Dr. Ito found that:

(1) Reishi reinforces membrane integrity of the cancerous

cell that impedes spreading (metastasis).

(2) Reishi prevents blood clot formation.

(3) Using Reishi in addition to other anti-tumor drugs and chemotherapy diminishes their side-effects and enhances their effect.

(4) It normalizes overall body function and, in turn, reduces the number of complications from treatment.

While we know that mushroom extracts have regulating effects and/or anti-tumor activity, the standard scientific approach has been to isolate, analyze, and administer the pure active components in any testing that's done. But different components in a mushroom extract can have activities that can work together. There are several reports of mushrooms containing more than one polysaccharide with anti-tumor activity. The responses of the tumor to different polysaccharides are likely to be the result of different cell surface receptors, which may be present only on specific subsets of cells and may trigger distinct downstream responses.

A combination of such responses involving different cell subsets could conceivably provide greater tumor inhibition than could be induced by a single polysaccharide. It is important to take a Red Reishi supplement as opposed to taking it's components in isolation.

In nature, synergy is always king!

"I started using Red Reishi essence (started 7 days prior) before my last Chemo (March 12th) and can attest the fact that I seemed to have additional energy and less side affects.

I can advise that, unless I am "dreaming", I definitely have increased energy (walking 3 km most days and doing many chores around home which I have not done since last summer) and according to others who have seen me with my prior Chemos, I have better colour and an upbeat attitude. I had a blood test a week ago and ALL my counts are in the healthy normal range. I used to lie down in the evenings after dinner because I was tired and since I have been using 2 caps per day I only rested once since my last Chemo.

John O.- retired businessman

FREQUENTLY ASKED QUESTIONS

IS RED REISHI SAFE TO TAKE WITH OTHER SUPPLEMENTS OR PRESCRIPTION MEDICATIONS?

To date, there are no known counter indications with taking Red Reishi alongside other supplements or prescriptions. However, if you are unsure, you should consult a medical practitioner who has an understanding of Reishi for use in complimentary care.

HOW LONG SHOULD I TAKE RED REISHI FOR?

Red Reishi is best taken as a daily supplement to maintain the benefits and your health long-term. It is safe to take on a continuous basis as part of a healthy lifestyle program.

WHEN SHOULD I TAKE IT?

For optimal results it is best to take Red Reishi first thing in the morning, with Vitamin C and plenty of water. If you forget at that time, it is still ok to take it later in the day when you can.

WHY IS VITAMIN C IMPORTANT?

Studies have shown that taking Red Reishi with a source of Vitamin C further enhances absorption and amplifies its effectiveness.

ARE THERE ANY SIDE EFFECTS?

No, there are no side effects from taking Red Reishi. In rare cases, some extra sensitive individuals do experience mild detoxification symptoms for the first few days of taking a Red Reishi supplement. Though unlikely, these may include slight itchiness, mild digestive upset, or changes in bowel movements. These symptoms usually disappear on their own within a couple of days, once the body has rid itself of its accumulated toxins. If they persist longer, consult your health care advisor.

QUALITY MATTERS

Choosing the Right Red Reishi Product

There are 2000 known species of Reishi, but the most important ones are identified by their colour: Black, Blue, White,
Yellow, Purple and Red. These are the species that have been
most closely studied. Of all of these, the Red variety is the
most commonly cultivated, because it has been found to be
the most effective; however, variations in the way the mushrooms are grown and harvested can make large differences
in the quality of the end product.

So, let's talk for a moment about the way that Red Reishi
supplements are produced, and what you need to know to
help you make the best choice of products on the market.

**First, you should be sure that the Red Reishi you are
buying has been cultivated, and is not collected in the
wild.** In addition to wide variation in the quality of mushrooms found naturally, due to variable growing conditions,
Red Reishi is often found in environmentally sensitive areas.
Collecting it may be causing damage to these areas.

As a result, the majority of Red Reishi products on the
market today use mushrooms that have been cultivated in
hothouses. Cultivation of Red Reishi originated in Gunma-
Ken, Japan, where the Mayuzumi family mastered the technique of culturing Red Reishi on Japanese Oak logs.

In addition, most of the Reishi that is sold as "wild" is of the
Black variety. While this variety has some benefit as a tonic,

Red Reishi has a much higher polysaccharide concentration, and is therefore more effective.

Secondly, some Reishi products are simply pulverized mushroom powder with bulk fillers – and often with cheap bulk fillers. You should be aware that these types of products are largely ineffective. Since the mushroom body contains a substance called chitin (KITE-in), they are rather wood-like in texture. For this reason, they are too tough and indigestible to be fully absorbed by the body unless they are further processed into an extract. Also note that the ground mushroom particles themselves are separate from the medically active ingredients – they do not contribute to strength and can cause an allergic reaction in some people. Always be sure to **look for a Red Reishi product that is in essence/extract form to ensure total bioavailability and results!** The best quality products are essence in a granular or capsule form.

The biggest consideration, though, is the technique that is used to cultivate the plant, and how it is processed. As we said earlier, Red Reishi is very hard to grow and that's the reason that it was so rare for so long. The plant will only grow in specific conditions that occur very infrequently in nature, and it's also sensitive to pollution, disease, and insects. Not many wild Red Reishi reach full, maximum potency and maturity. Reishi spores are very tough, and, in nature, they must land on decaying trees of just the right type, in just the right conditions of temperature, moisture, and light to grow. Red Reishi is so rare, that out of 10,000 such aged trees, only 2 or 3 will have Reishi growth; therefore, its wild form is rarely found.

As you can imagine, it took many years of research to understand exactly what conditions result in a healthy, mature Red Reishi. Japanese growers were the first to perfect these impeccable standards of Red Reishi cultivation and extraction. To this day, the quality of the Japanese Red Reishi's medicinal value is unsurpassed.

Research has proven that it is best to harvest only fully mature plants. In these plants, concentrations of the health-enhancing compounds are greatest, and the extract that results is most effective. Many methods used to cultivate Red Reishi result in small, immature plants with less than maximum efficiency. For this reason, not all of the Reishi products on the market are the same.

Common Growing Techniques

Common growing techniques used in North America, China, Malaysia, Korea and Vietnam include cultivation in glass or plastic containers and wood boxes. These methods are very inexpensive – the containers can be stacked in warehouses and no nutrient-rich soil is used.

To get a high turnover rate of crop, the reishi are often left to grow for as little as 3 to 5 months. The combination of no soil and a short growing period, renders a reishi crop with very low levels of phytonutrients. At this stage many companies simply grind up the dried reishi mushrooms and put them in capsules. Supplements that are composed of pulverized reishi powder are difficult for the body to absorb, and fewer results can be expected from taking them.

Common Growing Methods

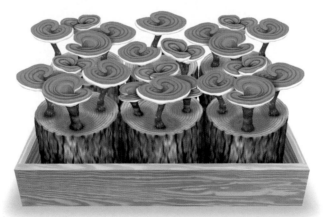

WOODEN BOX CULTIVATION METHOD

Grown 3 to 5 months; mid-size mushrooms;
no soil; low nutrient content

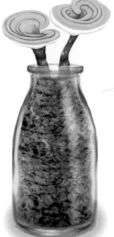

WOOD PULP/PAPER CULTIVATION IN GLASS OR PLASTIC CONTAINERS

Grown up to 3 months; no soil; very low nutritional content

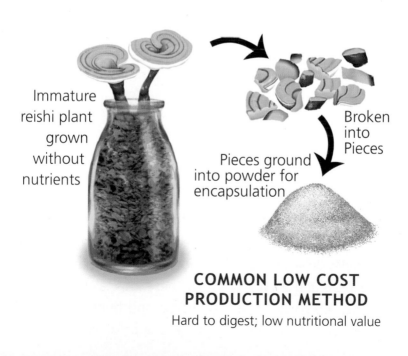

Immature reishi plant grown without nutrients

Broken into Pieces

Pieces ground into powder for encapsulation

COMMON LOW COST PRODUCTION METHOD

Hard to digest; low nutritional value

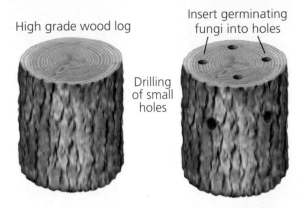

High grade wood log

Drilling of small holes

Insert germinating fungi into holes

Japanese woodlogs are drilled with holes
before mycelium are placed into it

The Japanese secret for superior Red Reishi cultivation

Until 30 years ago, the rare Red Reishi mushroom could only be found in nature. The cultivation of Red Reishi was considered impossible until a scientific breakthrough occurred in Japan due to to the diligent work of Japanese researchers. It was then that a third generation mycologist and one of the pioneers in Reishi cultivation, Fumimaru Mayuzumi, developed the "natural wood log cultivation" method - it is still considered today as the best way to produce high grade Red Reishi. This is the most complex form of cultivation, and takes almost a year to produce mature, potent plants.

Red Reishi spores from high quality mother plants, are cultured for three months in carefully controlled conditions, and then placed in holes drilled into selected high-grade logs that must be between 26 and 30 years of age. These logs, along with their spores, are placed in a greenhouse and buried under nutrient-rich soil for five months. It takes approximately five

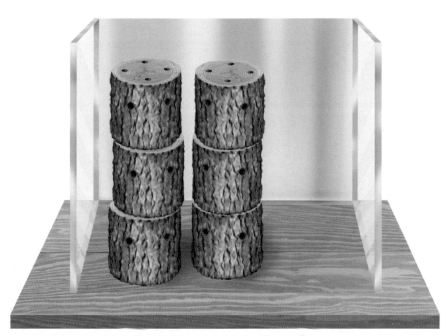

Woodlogs are placed in greenhouses for inoculation

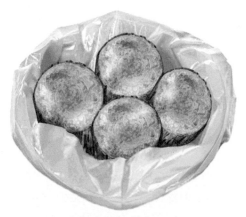

Inoculation Period

WOOD LOG WITH GERMINATING FUNGI REISHI

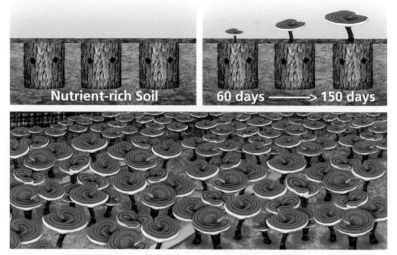

Japanese Red Reishi takes almost a full year
to get to the harvest stage!

months for the Red Reishi to absorb as many nutrients from the soil as it can. This soil is only used for five years. After that, it is left to recover nutrients for two to three years.

During the time that the crop is in the greenhouse soil, it is very closely monitored for temperature, humidity (between 90-95 percent), nutrients, carbon dioxide, and light intensity. It's an extremely painstaking process. The beds are sprayed daily with sanitized water to prevent bacterial infection. Soil nutrients are also monitored very closely to eliminate any natural metals, inert toxins, heavy metals, pollutants, or other contaminants. After this time, they are left to mature for yet another three-month period. Eventually they produce a thick coating of spores, and spraying is stopped when the spores are released into the air. The Reishi are allowed to mature another two weeks after the spores are released, and then harvested.

SUPERIOR QUALITY JAPANESE RED REISHI

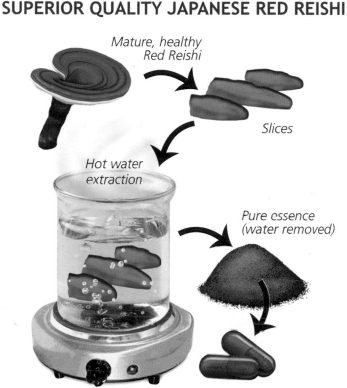

Mature, healthy Red Reishi

Slices

Hot water extraction

Pure essence (water removed)

100% bio-available essence encapsulated

After harvesting, the mushrooms are cut into small pieces, and boiled for several hours. This process is repeated three times to completely extract the Red Reishi essence, which not only contains the highest levels of the medicinal extracts, but is also in the most bio-available form.

This medicinal extract is prepared using a low temperature vacuum condenser and an air-spray dryer to transform it from a concentrated liquid, to a powder. The powder is then placed into certified vegetarian capsules and packaged. Strict control of moisture and temperature during the drying process is necessary to ensure high quality. This process of extraction also removes any residue of mushroom plant fibers that may cause an allergic reaction.

This method, while being much more expensive and time-consuming than some others, has been shown to produce the most effective, consistently high quality, medical grade products in essence form. In addition, it results in supplements that do not contain any mushroom fibers that might cause an allergic reaction. Some people who are normally allergic to mushrooms experience no adverse reaction when they take high quality Japanese Red Reishi in essence form.

Reishi Spores and Mycelium

The effectiveness of using the fruiting body of Red Reishi mushrooms in health supplements has made many companies eager to exploit other aspects of the Reishi mushroom for use in health products.

Recently, there has been much debate about the issue of whether supplements prepared by extracting oil from Reishi spores have more medicinal value than traditional Red Reishi products. In the past, the oxidation of Reishi oil was shown to create an unpleasant odor and become harmful to human cells. However, current marketers of these Reishi spore oil products claim to have perfected the technology of cracking the spores and preventing the lipid oil collected from being spoiled by oxidation.

The Hong Kong Consumer Council's* Choice magazine has thus far declined to comment on the medical efficacy of Reishi spore byproducts, stating that consumers should wait for more scientific research and clinical studies on these products before making a decision.

Mycelium

Another recent trend in the Reishi industry is the use of mycelium in place of mature Reishi mushroom extract in certain products. Mycelium is the stage between the spore and the mature mushroom in the Reishi life cycle. Reishi mycelium products are typically produced by mixing a small amount of mycelium with sterilized soybeans, rice, or other grains in a water slurry. The resulting mixture is then dried and ground into a powder for use in tablets of capsules.

While mycelium may possess some health-enhancing properties, specialists point out that all the research conducted thus far has centered on the various health benefits provided by the Reishi mushroom itself, and not the mycelium. Therefore, similar to the situation concerning spore oil products, there is currently insufficient evidence to support the claim that mycelium-based products can yield the same benefits as products made with the Red Reishi's fruiting body.

While mycelium use has become prevalent in North America, the lack of time-tested cultivation techniques for the substance has resulted in most mycelium cultivation to take place in greenhouses, using nutrients of less-than-optimum quality.

* The Consumer Council was established in April 1974 in Hong Kong. The function of the Council is to protect and promote the interests of consumers of goods and services and purchasers of immovable property. Some objectives of the Council are to conduct tests, surveys and research for the evaluation of goods and services to users; promote public awareness of consumer rights and responsibilities through publicity and media campaigns; and publish a monthly magazine "Choice" for the provision of independent and objective consumer information.

Growing Reishi mycelium in vats of grain slurry is considerably faster and cheaper than taking the Reishi mycelium through the next stage of growth to produce natural mature mushrooms. In contrast, growing mature Reishi mushrooms from mycelium requires 6 to 8 additional months in larger, shaded greenhouses equipped with sophisticated sterility, temperature, and humidity controls. Many producers find the additional cost and time necessary to organically cultivate the Reishi to maturity by this method too costly, and opt for the cheaper vat method, which may dilute the mycelium's potency, if any.

Although this cost-cutting practice is widely accepted in America, it is looked upon with disdain in China and Japan; to this day, companies in both countries where Reishi use has the longest history refuse to use mycelium in health products.

Consumers who are interested in using products derived from either Reishi spore oil or mycelium are advised to carefully research these topics, and consult a qualified health care professional before consuming any such products.

> *"I am very sensitive to my immune system and I noticed that my blood pressure was more stable, my energy levels were more even (I usually experience a 3:00 pm low - this energy stability happened gradually over a few days) and I had a general feeling of well-being. I should add that I am normally allergic to mushrooms, but probably because this is an extraction, rather than the mushroom itself, I had no adverse reaction."*
> Olga O.- personal shopper

Be Sure You Are Getting the Best!

WHAT TO LOOK FOR:

- **Red Reishi** (not just reishi or black reishi)
- **Essence/extract products**
  (not pulverized, ground or powdered)
- Capsules should be a **dark reddish brown colour**
- If you opened the capsule and tasted the essence, it should be very **bitter** (bitter means better!)
- Look for **Japan Reishi Association** (JRA) hologram on the package to ensure quality and country of origin (see page 92 for further details)

CONCLUSION

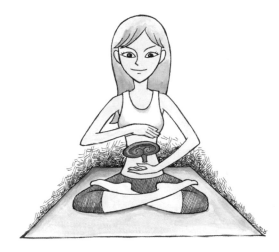

IT'S REALLY EXCITING TO THINK ABOUT THE MANY WAYS that Japanese Red Reishi can improve our overall health. It helps in the treatment of many diseases, works hard to help detoxify our bodies and fights the aging process; it also helps to protect us from pollutants we ingest and breathe everyday.

Life is stressful and can zap our energy, deplete our resources and set us up for disease. It's up to each one of us to be proactive, to stay strong and to function at our best. We have "many miles to go before we sleep" and there are many people who depend on us and love us.

Taking Japanese Red Reishi is an excellent way to help to keep your body and mind strong and in balance. It has been used successfully for thousands of years; it has been an important symbol of health and prosperity since ancient times and now, we are fortunate that this incredible herb is finally available here in North America. You've read the research, now you can make an informed choice to protect and preserve your health and vitality. Enjoy the natural healing properties of Japanese Red Reishi essence with no side effects. Make Japanese Red Reishi an important part of your daily health regime –you will be amazed at how great you can feel!

"To live is the rarest thing in the world. Most people exist, that is all." - Oscar Wilde

Looking for More Information?

Contact the Japan Reishi Association (JRA)

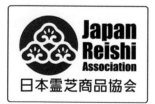

The Japan Reishi Association is an international nonprofit organization supported by industry leaders dedicated to helping growers and manufacturers maintain the highest standards of product quality and business practices in the Reishi industry worldwide.

The JRA's primary goal is to inform the general public about Reishi, Reishi-related health food products, and product manufacturers. In addition, the JRA is also committed to holding manufacturers and marketers of Reishi products accountable for claims of Japanese origin. To this end the JRA strives to set and aid in the enforcement of industry standards for product quality and ethical business practices by working together with authentic Reishi product manufacturers in Japan and international government organizations to alert the public about products and manufacturers that fail to meet these standards.

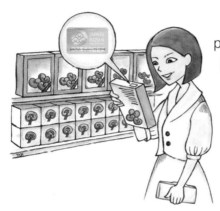

To verify you are purchasing an authentic, high-quality reishi product of Japanese origin--be sure to look for the Japan Reishi Association hologram logo on the package. If you have any questions about a Reishi product or manufacturer (such as the authenticity of a specific product you have purchased) you can contact the Japan Reishi Association at info@japan-reishi.org, or by calling their toll free number at 1-866-573-4744 in North America.

About the Authors:

Brad King, M.Sc., MFS, is a Canadian-based nutritional researcher, performance nutritionist and fitness expert who holds a Master's degree in nutritional science, and is certified by the International Sports Sciences Association as a Master of fitness science and a specialist in performance nutrition. Aside from authoring ten books, including the international best-seller, Fat Wars, Brad also writes the monthly newsletter Awaken Your Body with Brad King and the popular monthly Metabolism Matters column for Canada's #1 health magazine, Alive. Brad has spent the last decade researching and developing leading-edge dietary supplements and exercise protocols designed to improve health, slow biological aging, boost athletic performance, aid in fat loss and reduce excess inflammation. He is a highly sought after nutritional consultant and spokesperson, who has worked with nutritional companies across North America formulating numerous gold medal winning nutritional formulas. Brad sits on the scientific advisory board for the Fat Loss Research Institute, the Sports Nutrition Advisor Certification Course, and is a 2003 inductee into the prestigious Canadian Sports Nutrition Hall of Fame. Brad has been highlighted in numerous national magazines, health publications and newspapers and has appeared as a leading health and fitness expert on hundreds of national television programs in both Canada and the U.S., including The Today Show, Canada AM, Balance TV, Cityline, Body and Health and has also been a featured expert on over a thousand radio talk shows across North America. For more information please visit: www.AwakenYourBody.com

Dr. Meg Jordan, PhD, RN, is a medical anthropologist, an international health journalist, registered nurse, editor and founder of American Fitness Magazine, and on faculty at two universities, San Francisco State University and California Institute of Integral Studies. Known as the Global Medicine Hunter®, she searches the world for healing remedies. As a clinician at the Health Medicine Center in northern California, she specializes in behavioral health. She hosts the weekly morning newscast "Healthy Living" for Global TV, and hosts a daily radio program, (The Dr. Meg Jordan Show) on Health Radio Network. A former health reporter for FOX in San Francisco and a regular commentator for CNN, her columns have appeared in over 800 newspapers. She has authored several books in health and fitness, including The Fitness Instinct, and the upcoming Adventures of a Global Medicine Hunter. Meg serves on numerous advisory boards, including the National Wellness Institute and the Aerobics and Fitness Association of America, and is a recipient of awards such as the Healthy American Fitness Leader and the National Wellness Institute Service and Leadership Circle. She enjoys time with family and friends, racing sailboats, traveling the world, and hiking in redwood forests with her dog Kolya.

www.megjordan.com

REFERENCES

Aiko M, et al; Angiotensin Converting Enzyme-inhibitory Triterpenes from Ganoderma lucidum; Chem and Pharm Bulletin 37(2): 531-533 (1986)

Anderson RN, Smith BL. Deaths: leading causes for. Natl Vital Stat Rep. 2005 Mar 7;53(17):1-89 (2002).

Baillie-Hamilton PF. Chemical toxins: a hypothesis to explain the global obesity epidemic. J Altern Complement Med. Apr;8(2):185-92 (2002).

Bass, L, Young, A. The Dietary Supplement Health and Education Act: A Legislative History and Analysis Washington D.C. Food and Drug Law Institute (1996).

Borchers AT, Keen CL, Gershwin ME. Mushrooms, tumors, and immunity: an update. Exp Biol Med(Maywood). 229(5):393–406 (2004).

Bjorntorp P, Rosmond R. Neuroendocrine abnormalities in visceral obesity. Int J Obes Relat Metab Disord Jun; 24 Suppl 2:S80-5 (2000).

Brain, Behavior, and Immunity 18 114–119, http://psychology.uchicago.edu/people/faculty/cacioppo/jtcreprints/hc04.pdf (2004)

Chang HM, But RPH. "Lingzhi". In Pharmacology and Application of Chinese Materia Medica, Vol. I. World Scientific: Singapore, 642, 1986.

Chang, R. Effective Dose of Ganoderma in Humans; Proceedings of Contributed Symposium 59A, B 5th International Mycological Congress, Vancouver: pp. 117-121 (1994)

Chang, R. Limitations and Potential applications of Ganoderma and related fungal polyglycans in clinical ontology; First International Conference on Mushroom Biology and Mushroom products: 96 (1993)

Chen, A. W., et al. Ecological Studies of a long-spores Ganoderma species from the Savannah river site, South Carolina; First International Conference on Mushroom Biology and Mushroom products: 103 (1993)

Corrada, M., et al. Nonsteroidal anti-inflammatory drugs and the risk of Alzheimers disease. Neurology, 46, A433 (1996).

Diabesity® is a registered trademark of Shape Up America!

Effros RB. Replicative senescence of CD8 T cells: effect on human ageing. Exp Gerontol. Apr;39(4):517-24 (2004)

Effros RB, et al. The role of CD8+ T-cell replicative senescence in human aging. Immunol Rev. Jun;205:147-57 (2005).

Epel ES, et al. Accelerated telomere shortening in response to life stress. Proc Natl Acad Sci U S A. Dec 7;101(49):17312-5 (2004).

Gibson EL. Emotional influences on food choice: sensory, physiological and psychological pathways. Physiol Behav. Aug 30;89(1):53-61 (2006).

Golik A, et al. Elevated serum liver enzymes in obesity: a dilemma during clinical trials. Int J Obes. Dec;15(12):797-801 (1991).

Hikino H, et al. Mechanisms of Hypoglycemic Activity of Ganoderan B: A Glycan of Ganoderma lucidum Fruit Bodies. Planta Med. Oct;55(5):423-28 (1999).

Jung K, , et al. Antiviral effect of Saccharomyces cerevisiae beta-glucan to swine influenza virus by increased production of interferon-gamma and nitric oxide. J Vet Med B Infect Dis Vet Public Health. Mar;51(2):72-6 (2004).

Kenneth J. REISHI: Ancient herb for modern times. Sylvan Press, 1992.

Oliver G, et al. Stress and food choice: a laboratory study. Psychosom Med. Nov;62(6):853-65 (2000).

Maseri, A. Inflammation, atherosclerosis, and ischemic events-exploring the hidden side of the moon. New England J Medicine, 336 (14) 1014-1015 (1997)

Kadyrova RKh, et al. Effect of diet therapy using horse meat on liver function of patients with metabolic-alimentary obesity. Vopr Pitan. May-Jun;(3):22-7 (1984).

Katsuo Kanmatsue, et al; Studies on Ganoderma lucidum. Ffficacy against Hypertension and Side Effects; Yakugako Zasshi 105(10): 942-947 (1985)

King, B. Fat Wars: 45 Days to Transform Your Body (updated edition). Toronto: CDG Books Canada Inc., 2002.

Komorovskii IuT, et al. Liver function in patients with obesity. Vrach Delo. May;(5):83-5 (1978)

Lakshmi, T.A., et al. Antiperoxidative, anti-inflammatory, and antimutagenic activities of ethanol extract of the mycelium of Ganoderma lucidum occur-ring in South India. Teratog-Carcinog-Mutagen. 23 Suppl 1: 85-97 (2003)

Li Guangzhou. Anti-tumor function about polysaccharide of mushroom. Chinese Journal of Modern Applied Medicine. 17(5):354-355 (2000)

Marin, P., et al. "Cortisol Secretion in Relation to Body Fat Distribution in Obese Premenopausal Women." Metabolism 41, no. 8, Aug :882–886 (1992).

McGeer, P., & Rogers, J. Anti-inflammatory agents as a therapeutic approach to Alzheimers disease. Neurology, 42, 447-449 (1992).

McTernan CL, et al. Resistin, central obesity, and type 2 diabetes.Lancet. Jan 5;359(9300):46-7 (2002).

Michihiro K., et al. "Immuno-potentiating Effects of the Antler-shaped Fruiting Body of Ganoderma lucidum (Rokkaku-Reishi)", Biosci. Biotechnol. Biochem., Vol. 68, 881-887 (2004).

Minino AM, et al. Deaths: preliminary data for 2004. Natl Vital Stat Rep. Jun 28;54(19):1-49 (2006).

Mizuno, T. Oriental Medicinal tradition of Ganoderma lucidum (Reishi) in China. In T. Mizuno & B. -K. Kim (Eds.), Ganoderma lucidum (pp.101-106). Seoul, Korea: Il-Yang Pharm. Co. Ltd (1996).

Nagano, Y., Kojima,Y. "Inhibition de l'infection vaccinale par un facteur liquide dans le tissu infecté par le virus homologue" C.R. Seances Soc. Biol. Fil. 152:1672-1629 (1958)

Nomura F, et al. Liver function in moderate obesity--study in 534 moderately obese subjects among 4613 male company employees. Int J Obes. 10(5):349-54 (1986).

Ohe K, et al. Obesity and liver dysfunction in UOEH employees--multiple regression analysis of the annual physical checkup data of 1991, J UOEH. Mar 1;17(1):11-29 (1995).

Pelletier, Kenneth. Mind as Healer, Mind as Slayer. New York: Delta, 1992

Ravaglia G. Determinants of functional status in healthy Italian nonagenarians and centenarians: a comprehensive functional assessment by the instruments of geriatric practice. J Am Geriatr Soc. Oct;45(10):1196-202 (1997)

Ridker, P.M, et al. Inflammation, aspirin, and the risk of cardiovascular disease in apparently healthy men. New England J. Medicine, 336 (14) 973-979 (1997)

Rogers, J.Inflammation as a pathogenic mechanism in Alzheimers disease. Arzheim. -Forsch., 45, 439-442 (1995)

Rosmond, R, et al. 5-HT2A Receptor Gene Promoter Polymorphism in Relation to Abdominal Obesity and Cortisol Obesity Research 10:585-589 (2002)

Stavinoha, WB., et al. Study of the antiinflammatory efficacy of Ganoderma lucidum. (1995).

Stengler, M, Prescription for Natural Cures. Wiley, (2005).

Steppan CM, et al. The hormone resistin links obesity to diabetes. Nature. Jan 18;409(6818):307-12 (2001).

The Gathering Storm: The Pre-Diabetes Epidemic. Nutrition Action Health Letter. June, Vol.31 #5 (2004)

Turkoglu C, et al. Effect of abdominal obesity on insulin resistance and the components of the metabolic syndrome: evidence supporting obesity as the central feature. Obes Surg. Oct;13(5):699-705 (2003).

Understanding the Immune System http://www.niaid.nih.gov/publications/immune/the_immune_system.pdf

http://en.wikipedia.org/wiki/White_blood_cell

Van der Hem, Van der Vliet, Kino, Hoitsma and Tax. Ling Zhi-8: A fungal protein with immunomodulatory effects Transplant. Proc. 28 (2); 958-959 (1996)

Vickers A. Botanical medicines for the treatment of cancer: rationale, overview of current data, and methodological considerations for phase I and II trials. Cancer Invest. 20(7-8):1069–1079 (2002).

Xiao Z, et al. Beta-glucan enhancement of T cell IFNgamma response in swine. Vet Immunol Immunopathol. Dec 8;102(3):315-20 (2004).

Yearul K., et al; Dietary Effect of Ganoderma lucidum Mushroom on Blood Pressure and Lipid Levels in Spontaneous Hypertensive Rats; Journal of Nutritional Science and Vitaminology 34(4): 433-438 (1988).

Zhang HN et al / Acta Pharmacol Sin Feb; 25 (2): 191-195 (2004)